DASH

DIET

Dash Diet for Every Day: The Ultimate Guide to Lower Your Blood Pressure With Change Your Eating Habits to Lower Your Blood Pressure and Lose Weight

@ Lynn Kim

Published By Adam Gilbin

@ Lynn Kim

Dash Diet for Every Day: The Ultimate Guide to Lower Your Blood Pressure With Change Your Eating Habits to Lower Your Blood Pressure and Lose Weight

All Right RESERVED

ISBN 978-1-990053-32-0

TABLE OF CONTENTS

Pear-Cranberry Pie With Oatmeal Streusel

Ingredients:

Streusel:

- 1 cup of regular oats
- 1   teaspoon of ground cinnamon
- 1/2 teaspoon of ground nutmeg
- 1 light brown sugar (packed)
- 1 tbsp unsalted butter (Chilled and small pieces)

Filling:

- 2 cups of fresh cranberries
- 3 cups (a 1 -inch) cubed (peeled /unpeeled) and 2 large pears
- 1   cup light brown sugar (packed)
- 2   tablespoons of cornstarch

Directions:

1. Preheat the oven to 350 °F.

2. Combine the first 4 ingredients in a medium bowl to cook streusel; cut into butter with a pastry cutter or 2 knives till the mixture is comparable to a coarse meal.

3. Combine cranberries, 2/3 cup of brown sugar, corn starch and pear in a wide bowl to prepare the filling. So mix well to combine. Sprinkle streusel over pear mixture and spoon the pear mixture into pastry shell.

4. Cook for 1 hour at 350 degrees or it is creamy, and streusel is browned.

5. Cool it on a wire rack for at least 1 hour.

Chef Roblé Ali's Homemade Guacamole

Ingredients:

- 1 cup scallions (chopped)
- 1/2 cup tomatoes (diced)
- 1 caustic lime (cut in 1)
- 1 clove garlic (chopped)
- pinch of cumin
- pinch of coriander
- pinch of chili powder
- 2 avocados

Directions:

1. Scoop and mash the avocado into a bowl.
2. Add other ingredients and mix well and serve.

Vegetable Pasta Soup

Ingredients:

- 2 tablespoons fresh parsley (snipped)

- 1 cup Parmesan cheese (shaved)

- 1 cup celery (thinly sliced)

- 1 cup onion (chopped)

- 25 ounce box chicken broth (reduced-sodium)

- 3 cups ditalini pasta (dried)

- 3 cups coarsen carrot (shredded)

- 12 (3/4-cup) appetizer servings

- 6 cloves minced garlic

- 4 cups of water

- 2 teaspoons of olive oil

Directions:

1. Heat the oil over medium heat in a 5 to 6 quart Dutch oven.

2. Combine with garlic; simmer for 15 seconds. Add the onion, carrot, and celery and then roast and stir regularly for 5 -7 min until it is tender.

3. Add the water and chicken broth and allow it to boil.

4. Stir in uncooked pasta and boil for 5 to 10 mins or until it is tender.

5. Cover individual pieces of parsley and Parmesan cheese to eat.

6. Allows 12 servings of (3/4-cup) appetizer.

Jamika Pessoa's Thai Peanut Salad

Ingredients:

- 1 cup lumpy peanut butter

- 1/2 teaspoon fresh/ground ginger

- 1/2 cup of cilantro leaves

- 1 tablespoon h2   y

- 1 cup chicken (shredded)

- 1 bag cabbage and carrot mix (shredded)

- Kosher salt & black pepper (cracked)

- juice & zest (1   a lime)

- 3 tablespoons of soy sauce

- 3 scallions (sliced)

- 2 tablespoon water (if needed to thin)

- 2 tablespoon rice or apple cider vinegar

Directions:

1. Put the cabbage in a serving bowl with the scallions, carrots, cilantro and chicken.
2. In a small cup, combine the remaining ingredients and whisk until combined.
3. Over the salad, pour the dressing and serve.

Easy Beef Brisket

Ingredients:

- Onions (chopped) 1 cups

- Garlic (peel and smash) 4 cloves

- Dried thyme 1 teaspoon

- Tomatoes and liquid (no salt added) 1 can (14.5 ounces)

- Red wine vinegar 1 cup

- Beef stock (low-sodium) 1 cup

- Olive oil 1 tablespoon

- Beef brisket 2 pounds

- Black pepper (coarsely ground) as per taste

Directions:

1. Begin by trimming the fat off the beef brisket. Cut the brisket into 8 equal-sized pieces.

2. Preheat the oven by setting the temperature to 350 degrees Fahrenheit.

3. Place the brisket pieces in a shallow dish and sprinkle with coarsely ground pepper.
4. Make sure the brisket is evenly coated.
5. Take a large-sized Dutch oven and place it on a medium-high flame.
6. Pour in a tablespoon of oil and let it heat through.
7. Add the seas 2 brisket pieces to the Dutch oven and cook until the meat turns dark brown on each side.
8. This will take about 5 to 10 minutes.
9. Turn every 2 minutes to prevent the meat from burning.
10. Once d2 , transfer the brisket onto a plate and set it aside.
11. Add the onion to the Dutch oven and sauté until it begins to caramelize.
12. Also, add in the thyme and garlic and sauté for around a minute.

13. Now add in the tomatoes and the juice, beef stock, and vinegar.

14. Mix well and let it come to a boil.

15. Return the sautéed beef brisket to the Dutch oven and cook with tomatoes and stock mixture for about 18 hours or until the beef is tender.

16. Serve hot!

Spiced Chipotle Shrimp

Ingredients:

- Fresh oregano (chopped) 1 teaspoon
- Shrimp (uncooked; peeled and deveined) 1 pound
- Tomato paste 2 tablespoons
- Water 1 teaspoons
- Olive oil (extra-virgin) 1 teaspoon
- Garlic (minced) 1 teaspoon
- Chipotle chili powder 1 teaspoon

Directions:

1. Begin by rinsing the shrimp in cold running water.
2. Use a kitchen paper towel to pat the shrimp dry and set it aside.
3. Take a shallow dish and fill it 1 way with water.

4. Place the skewers into the same to soak.

5. To prepare the marinade, take a small glass bowl and add in the tomato paste, oil, and water.

6. Use a whisk to combine all the ingredients well.

7. Also, add in the chili powder, oregano, and garlic. Whisk well.

8. Use a baking brush to coat both sides of the shrimp with the marinade and place them in the fridge for about 1 an hour.

9. Prepare the charcoal grill by lighting the fire. Take the grill rack and lightly grease it with cooking spray. Place the grill rack about 6 inches above the fire.

10. Insert the marinated shrimp into the skewers and place it onto the greased grill rack. Grill for 3 minutes; flip over and grill for another 3 minutes.

11. Transfer onto a serving platter and serve right away!

Puttanesca Served With Brown Rice

Ingredients:

- Garlic (minced) 1 tablespoon

- Olive oil 1 tablespoon

- Fresh basil (chopped) 1/2 cup

- Fresh parsley (minced) 1 tablespoon

- Red pepper flakes 1/2 teaspoon

- Brown rice (cooked) 3 cups

- Plum tomatoes (chopped) 4 cups

- Kalamata olives (sliced) 4

- Green olives (sliced) 4

- Capers (rinsed and drained) 2 tablespoons

Directions:

1. Take a large glass mixing bowl and add in the chopped tomatoes, Kalamata olives, green olives, garlic, oil, and capers. Toss well.
2. Also, add in the parsley, red pepper flakes, and basil.
3. Toss until all ingredients are well combined. Cover the glass bowl with a lid or cling film and let it sit for 30 minutes at room temperature. Give it a toss every 10 minutes.
4. To serve, take a plate and place the rice into the same.
5. Top with prepared puttanesca. Serve!

Chicken Asparagus Penne

Ingredients:

- Tomatoes including juice (diced) 1 (5 ounces) can

- Dried oregano 2 teaspoons

- Soft goat cheese (crumbled) 1 tablespoon

- Parmesan cheese 1 tablespoon

- Penne pasta (whole-grain) 1 cups

- Asparagus 1 cup, cut into 1-inch pieces

- Chicken breasts (b2 less and skinless) 6 ounces, cut into 1-inch cubes

- Garlic (minced) 2 cloves

Directions:

1. Begin by cutting the asparagus into pieces measuring about an inch each.
2. Also, cut the chicken breasts into 1-inch cubes.

3. Take a large stockpot and fill it with water. Let it come to a boil.

4. Once the water begins to boil, add in the pasta and cook as per package instructions.

5. This will normally take about 10 to 15 minutes.

6. Once the pasta is al dente, drain into a colander and set aside.

7. Take a steamer and fill the steamer pot with water up to 1 inch in height.

8. Add the cut asparagus to the steamer basket and place it over the pot once the water comes to a boil. Cover with a lid and steam for around 3 minutes.

9. While the asparagus steams, take a large nonstick pan and place it on a medium-high flame. Grease it lightly with cooking spray.

10. Add the garlic and chicken to the pan and sauté for about 7 minutes. The chicken should be golden brown.

11. Add in the tomatoes along with the juice and oregano and cook for another 1 minute.

12. Stir well and remove from the flame.

13. Transfer the cooked pasta into a large glass mixing bowl along with the steamed asparagus and prepared chicken and tomato mixture.

14. Also, add in the crumbled goat cheese and give a nice toss. Make sure all ingredients are well combined.

15. Serve on pasta plates topped with a generous sprinkle of parmesan cheese.

16. Enjoy!

Asian-Style Grilled Salmon

Ingredients:

Sesame oil 1 tablespoon

Soy sauce (reduced-sodium) 1 tablespoon

Fresh ginger (minced) 1 tablespoon

Rice wine vinegar 1 tablespoon

Salmon fillets 4

Directions:

1. Take a shallow dish and add in the sesame oil, ginger, vinegar, and soy sauce. Mix well to combine.
2. Place the salmon fillets in the dish and flip over to coat both sides.
3. Place the marinated salmon into the fridge for around an hour.
4. Flip after every 15 minutes.

5. Prepare the grill by lighting the fire and lightly coat the grill rack with oil. Make sure the temperature is medium-high.

6. Place the marinated fish fillets on the rack and cook for 5 minutes on each side. Make sure the fish is no longer pink.

7. Serve warm!

Pork Medallions In Five Spices

Ingredients:

- Black pepper (freshly ground) 1 tablespoon

- Chicken stock (no salt added) 2 cups

- Chicken breasts (b2   less and skinless) 2

- Red beets (diced) 1 cup

- Butternut squash (peel and dice) 1 cup

- Beet tops greens (chopped) 2 cups

- Balsamic vinegar 1 tablespoon

- Dried cranberries 2 tablespoons

- Canola oil   1 tablespoon

- Carrots (sliced)   2 cups

- Yellow onion (diced)   1 cup

- Fresh mushrooms   1 cup

- Fresh parsley (minced)   2 tablespoons

- Fancy wild rice (uncooked)   1 cup

- Walnuts (chopped)   2 tablespoons

Directions:

1. Begin by heating a nonstick saucepan on a medium flame.

2. Pour in 1 tablespoon of oil and let it heat through.

3. Once hot, toss in the carrots, mushrooms, parsley, and onion.

4. Sauté for around 10 minutes or until they begin to caramelize.

5. Stir in the wild rice, chicken stock, walnuts, and black pepper; let it come to a boil and then reduce the flame. Cover the saucepan with a lid and cook for around 40 minutes.

6. While the rice is cooking, add the remaining 1 teaspoon of oil.

7. Once the oil is hot, place the chicken breasts into the same and cook for around 3 minutes on each side.

8. Once d2 , remove the chicken onto a plate and set it aside.

9. Add the squash and beets to the pan; stir well and cook for about 20 minutes. The squash should be tender by now.

10. Add the prepared rice mixture, balsamic vinegar, chopped greens, and cranberries to the pan. Stir until well combined.

11. To serve, transfer into a serving bowl and top with chicken breasts.

12. Serve right away!

Stuffed Baked Apples

Ingredients:

- Orange Zest (2 T)

- Dried Apricots (.4 C)

- Flaked Coconut (.4 C)

- Apples (4)

- Brown Sugar (2 T)

- Orange Juice (.50 C)

Directions:

1. First, you will want to prepare your apples.
2. You can do this by peeling the top third of the apple and then hollow out the centers.
3. Next, you will want to combine the apricots with the orange zest and the coconut.
4. When this is set, scoop it into the center of the apples.
5. In a small bowl, mix together the brown sugar and orange juice and then pour over the

apples that are placed in a microwave-safe
dish.

6. Pop the apples into your microwave for eight
minutes.

7. By the end of this time, the apples should be
soft.

8. Take the apples out, allow them to cool, and
then enjoy your dessert.

Creamy Apple Shake

Ingredients:

- Applesauce (1 C)

- Low-fat Vanilla Ice Cream (2 C)

- Fat-free Milk (1 C)

- Ground Cinnamon (.25 t)

Directions:

1. Making this creamy apple shake is super easy! First, stick all of the ingredients into a blender and mix until the shake becomes smooth.
2. Place your shake in a glass and serve.
3. For some extra flavor, sprinkle some cinnamon on top!

Watermelon Sorbet

Ingredients:

- Simple Sugar Syrup (1 C)

- Watermelon (8 C)

- Lemon Juice (2 T)

Directions:

1. Begin by placing the watermelon into a food processor and blend until it is smooth.
2. Next, add in the lemon juice and simple sugar syrup and blend for another few seconds.
3. Pour all of the ingredients into a small bowl and place in freezer.
4. Allow the mix to freeze for a few hours and then serve for a nice, refreshing dessert!

Egg Melts

Ingredients:

- 1/2 teaspoon sea salt, fine
- 1/2 teaspoon black pepper
- 1 cup swiss cheese, shredded & reduced fat
- 1 cup grape tomatoes, quartered
- 1 teaspoon olive oil
- english muffins, whole grain & split
- scallions, sliced fine
- 8 egg whites, whisked

Directions:

1. Set the oven to broil, and then put your english muffins on a baking sheet.
2. Make sure the split side is facing up.
3. Broil for 3   minutes. They should turn golden around the edges.

4. Get out a skillet and grease with oil. Place it over medium heat, and cook your scallions for three minutes.
5. Beat your egg whites with salt and pepper, and pour this over your scallions.
6. Cook for another minute, stirring gently.
7. Spread this on your muffins, and top with remaining scallions if desired, cheese and tomatoes.
8. Broil for 1 to 5 more minutes to melt the cheese and serve warm.

Fluffy Pancakes For Breakfast

Ingredients:

- Baking powder 1 teaspoon

- Baking soda 1/2 teaspoon

- White sugar 2 tablespoons

- Salt 1/2 teaspoon

- Cooking spray

- Eggs 1

- Melted butter 2 tablespoons

- White vinegar 2 tablespoons

- Milk 2 cup

- All-purpose flour 1 cup

Directions:

1. Begin with mixing milk and vinegar in a bowl and leave the solution for 5 minutes until it turns "sour".

2. Whip egg and butter together into the "soured" milk emulsion.

3. Add all-purpose flour, baking powder, baking soda, sugar, and salt in a separate bowl.

4. Take all the wet comp2   nt and mix with the flour emulsion.

5. Whisk the mixture until it becomes an even paste.

6. Take a frying pan and heat it over medium heat. Now coat the pan with cooking spray.

7. Take 1 cupful of the paste in a frying pan and cook well.

8. Use a spatula to flip the cake and cook until it turns fluffy and golden brown.

9. Transfer the pancakes onto a plate and garnish with your choice of cream.

Fluffy Zucchini Bread

Ingredients:

- Eggs 3

- Vegetable oil 1 cup

- Sugar 4 cups

- Vanilla extract 3 teaspoons

- Zucchini (grated) 2 cups

- Walnuts (chopped) 1 cup

- All-purpose white flour 3 cups

- Salt 1 teaspoon

- Baking soda 1 teaspoon

- Baking powder 1 teaspoon

- Cinnamon (ground) 1 teaspoon

Directions:

1. Start by preheating the oven to 350 degrees f (165 degrees c).

2. Now grease 3 9 x 5-inch pans or standard pans with cooking oil.

3. Flour the greased pans and remove the access flour.

4. Mix flour along with salt, baking powder, baking soda, and ground cinnamon.

5. In a separate bowl, take eggs, vegetable oil, sugar and vanilla extract and beat all the ingredients: together.

6. Add dry flour mixture in the creamed solution and beat until it becomes a thick paste.

7. Grate 3 cups of zucchini.

8. Add grated zucchini and chopped walnuts in the paste and stir until all the ingredients: are well combined in the flour paste.

9. Now pour the batter into the greased pans and bake for at least 40 to 60 minutes. Use a tester if required.

10. Let the bread cool in the pan until it is firm enough to be removed.

11. Cut into slices once the bread is completely cool.

Spinach Crestless Quiche

Ingredients:

- Eggs 5

- Muenster cheese (shredded) 3 cups

- Salt 1   teaspoon

- Black pepper (ground) 1 teaspoon

- Vegetable oil 1 tablespoon

- Chopped onion 1

- Frozen chopped spinach 10 ounce/1 package

Directions:

1. Begin with preheating the oven to 350 degrees f (175 degrees c).

2. Now grease a 9 x 5 inch pan or any standard pan with cooking oil.

3. Chop the onion and remove the frozen spinach in a strainer.

4. Squeeze spinach to remove all the extra moisture or water.
5. Heat vegetable oil in a large frying pan and add chopped onion into it.
6. Cook onions until they turn soft or light golden in color.
7. Add drained spinach into it and stir until moisture is evaporated and remover the mixture.
8. Take eggs in a fresh bowl and whip. Add salt, cheese, and pepper into it.
9. Now take the spinach mixture, add to the whipped egg solution, and stir until everything is blended well.
10. Pour mixture into the greased pan and bake in the oven for 30 minutes.
11. Leave the dish until it cools and serve by cutting into slices of your choice

Friendly French Toast

Ingredients:

- Cinnamon (ground) 1/2 teaspoon

- Vanilla extract 1 teaspoon

- Sugar 1 tablespoon

- Bread 12 slices

- All-purpose flour 1 cup

- Milk 1 cup

- Salt 1/2 teaspoon

- Eggs 3

Directions:

1. Take all-purpose flour in a bowl and add milk, eggs, salt (as per taste) and ground cinnamon, vanilla extract, and sugar.

2. Whisk the mixture to make a smooth paste.

3. Take a frying pan and heat it lightly.

4. Take a slice of bread and soak it completely in the paste. Repeat this with all the slices.
5. Now cook each slice of bread until it turns golden brown on both sides.
6. Serve hot with maple syrup.

Everyday Crepes

Ingredients:

- Water 1/2 cup

- Salt 1   teaspoon

- Butter (melted) 2 tablespoons

- All-purpose flour 1 cup

- Eggs 2

- Milk 1/2 cup

Directions:

1. Start by taking all-purpose flour in a mixing bowl and or milk, water, salt, eggs and whisk together to make a running paste.

2. Add melted butter to the paste.

3. Heat a frying pan on medium flame and add a quarter cup of the batter into it.

4. Spread the batter evenly in the frying pan and let the crepe cook on both the sides. Serve hot.

Hash Brown Cheesy Ham Casserole

Ingredients:

- Cream of potato soup (condensed) 2 cans

- Sour cream 1

- Cheddar cheese (shredded) 2 cups

- Parmesan cheese (grated) 2 cups

- Hash brown potatoes (frozen package) 1

- Diced ham (cooked) 8 ounces

Directions:

1. Start by preheating the oven to 375 degrees f (190 degrees c).

2. In a fresh bowl, take frozen packaged mix hash browns potatoes, diced cooked ham, shredded cheddar cheese, sour cream, and condensed cream of potato soup.

3. Mix all the ingredients: evenly. Now grease a large 9x13 inch baking dish and spread the mixture into it.

4. Sprinkle grated parmesan cheese to cover the mixture evenly in the baking dish.

5. Bake the dish in the oven for an hour until it is light brown in color.

6. Serve hot garnished with parmesan cheese

Scrambled Eggs With Hash Brown Potatoes

Ingredients:

- 1/2 cup chicken broth
- 1 whole egg
- 1 egg white
- 1 tablespoon fat-free milk
- 2 diced red-skin potatoes
- 1/2 diced yellow onion
- 1/2 diced green bell pepper
- Salt and pepper

Irections:

1. Pre-heat a skillet with olive oil and sauté potatoes, peppers and onions.
2. Season with salt and pepper and cook for about 10 minutes or until brown.

3. Add chicken broth and cook for 3 more minutes.

4. Blend the whole egg and egg white with fat-free milk. Mix well.

5. Stir the eggs into the vegetables and cook for about 20 minutes.

Stir-Fried Chicken And Brown Rice

Ingredients:

- 2 beaten eggs

- 3 cups cooked brown rice

- 2 minced garlic cloves

- 3 tablespoons peanut oil

- 1 teaspoon minced fresh ginger

- 1 pound sliced skinless and b2 less chicken thighs

- 4 tablespoons soy sauce

- 1 teaspoon cornstarch

- 3 minced scallions

Directions:

1. In a mixing bowl, combine scallions, cornstarch, soy sauce and chicken.

2. Marinate for 10 minutes.

3. Heat oil in a frying pan. Stir-fry ginger and garlic.

4. Add chicken and cook for 4 minutes. Remove the cooked chicken.

5. Use the same pan to cook the eggs. Dice the cooked eggs. Set aside.

6. Heat 1 tablespoon oil for 15 seconds in the same pan.

7. Use the same pan to stir fry the scallion and cooked rice.

8. Cook for 7 minutes. Add the eggs, chicken and soy sauce. Stir-fry for a minute. Serve hot.

Turkey Meatballs

Ingredients:

- 1 chopped green sweet pepper
- 2 minced garlic cloves
- cup rolled oats
- 1 beaten egg
- 1 teaspoon Creole seasoning
- 1 teaspoon salt-free seasoning blend
- 1 pound uncooked ground turkey
- 1 chopped onion
- tablespoons fat-free milk
- 1 teaspoon crushed dried Italian seasoning

Directions:

1. Preheat oven to 380 degrees Fahrenheit.
2. Grease a baking pan with cooking spray. Set aside.

3. Mix the sweet pepper, onion, egg, rolled oats, garlic and milk in a bowl.

4. Season with salt-free seasoning blend, Creole seasoning and Italian seasoning.

5. Add the turkey into the blend and mix well.

6. Mold the turkey mixture into balls.

7. Arrange the formed turkey balls into the baking pan.

8. Bake the turkey balls for about 25 minutes or until browned.

Shrimp, Beans And Carrots Stir-Fry

Ingredients:

- 8 sliced fresh greens

- 3 cup brown rice

- 1 pound fresh shrimp in shells

- 1 teaspoon chicken bouillon

- teaspoon dried dill

- 1 teaspoon shredded lemon peel

- julienned carrots

- 1 tablespoon butter

Directions:

1. Peel and devein shrimp. Leave tails intact.

2. Boil the brown rice in a saucepan for 40 minutes or until rice is tender.

3. Melt butter in a frying pan. Stir in the carrot and green beans for about 5 minutes.

4. In a mixing bowl, pour the water and bouillon granules.

5. Stir well until bouillon dissolves.

6. Add the water mixture, lemon peel, dill and deveined shrimp into the carrots and green beans in the frying pan.

7. Cook for 4 minutes uncovered. Serve hot.

Turkey Sausage And Potatoes

Ingredients:

- 4 tablespoons olive oil

- 1 teaspoons slightly crushed cumin seed

- 1 teaspoon crushed dried thyme

- Salt and pepper

- pound cooked smoked turkey sausage, sliced

- 1 pounds cubed red-skinned potato

- medium chopped onions

Directions:

1. Heat oil in an ovenproof pan.
2. Sauté the potatoes and onions for about 12 minutes.
3. Stir in the sausage into the potato mixture.
4. Cook for about 10 minutes or until the potatoes are slightly brown.
5. Add the thyme and cumin seed.

6. Season with salt and pepper.

Baked Halibut With Salsa

Ingredients:

- 1 teaspoon chopped fresh oregano

- 2 tablespoons chopped fresh basil

- 2 teaspoons extra-virgin olive oil

- 4 halibut fillets

- 2 diced tomatoes

- 1 tablespoon minced garlic

Directions:

1. Preheat oven to 350 degrees Fahrenheit.
2. Coat a baking pan with cooking spray.
3. Mix the basil, oregano, garlic and tomato in a mixing bowl. Add the olive oil.
4. Place the halibut fillet in the baking pan.
5. Top the tomato mixture over the fillet.
6. Bake for about 10 to 15 minutes.

Salad Sandwich

Ingredients:

- 2 slices multi-grain bread
- 1/2 peeled avocado
- 1/2 teaspoon lemon juice
- 1 slice cheddar cheese
- 2 tablespoons alfalfa sprouts
- 3 large slices ripe tomatoes
- 4 sliced peeled and seedless cucumber
- 1 tablespoon reduced-fat mayonnaise

Directions:

1. Spread the mayonnaise on each bread slice.
2. Mash the avocado and mix it with the lemon juice. Spread it over the mayonnaise.
3. Assemble the sandwich by topping with sprouts, tomatoes, cucumber and cheese.

Salsa Pizza

Ingredients:

- 2 cup chopped red or green bell peppers

- 2 cup seeded, peeled and chopped mango

- 1 cup chopped fresh cilantro

- 1 tablespoon lime juice

- 12-inch whole-grain pizza crust

- 2 cup minced onion

- 3 cup pineapple tidbits

Directions:

1. Preheat the oven to 450 degrees Fahrenheit. Coat a round baking pan with cooking spray.

2. Combine the mango, pineapple, lime juice, cilantro, peppers and onions in a mixing bowl. Set aside.

3. Bake the pizza dough in the oven for about 15 minutes.

4. Get the cooked pizza crust from the oven.

5. Spread the mango salsa over the crust.

6. Put it back into the oven and cook for about 10 minutes or until the crust is browned.

7. Slice the pizza into eight parts.

Pork Tenderloin In Fennel

Ingredients:

- 1 sliced fennel bulb

- 1 teaspoon fennel seeds

- 2 cup dry white wine

- 1 tablespoons olive oil

- 2 pork tenderloin fillets

- 1 can low-sodium chicken broth

- 1 sliced sweet onion

Directions:

1. Arrange pork between wax paper sheets. Pound the pork fillets with a mallet.

2. Heat oil over a pan. Put the fennel seeds and toast until fragrant.

3. Stir in the pork and cook for 3 minutes until browned. Set aside and keep warm.

4. Add the onion slices and fennel into the same pan. Sauté for about 5 minutes or until vegetables are tender. Set aside and keep warm.

5. Pour the wine and chicken broth to the same pan. Boil until reduced in 1 .

6. Put back the set aside pork into the pan and cook for 5 minutes.

7. Add the fennel and onion mixture and cook for about 3 more minutes.

Roasted Chicken With Rosemary And Orange Juice

Ingredients:

- 3 skinless chicken breast halves
- 1 teaspoons extra-virgin olive oil
- 3 teaspoons fresh rosemary
- Ground black pepper
- 2 minced garlic cloves
- 3 skinless chicken legs
- 1 cup orange juice

Directions:

1. Preheat the oven to 450 degrees Fahrenheit. Grease a baking pan with cooking spray.
2. Rub the chicken pieces with garlic, rosemary and pepper.
3. Place the herbed chicken on the baking pan.

4. Pour the orange juice over the chicken and bake for about 30 minutes.

Apple Muesli

Ingredients:

- 1 cup low-fat muesli with

- 1 cup fat-free milk

Directions:

1. Add diced apples, dried currants, raisins and cranberries. Sprinkle with cinnamon.

Orange And Banana Shake

Ingredients:

- 1 of a banana, 2   whole peeled orange

- 2 tablespoon h2   y

- 1/2 cup fat-free milk and 2 ice cubes.

Directions:

1. Add a dash of nutmeg.

2. Blend until smooth.

Shrimp Quesadillas

Ingredients:

- Combine 2 ounces low-fat smoked mozzarella cheese
- 1 teaspoon cumin
- 2 ounces diced cooked shrimp
- 1 deseeded and chopped tomato
- 1 diced jalapeño and 1/2 diced red onion in a mixing bowl.

Directions:

1. Spread the mixture over whole-wheat tortillas.
2. Heat the filled tortillas for about 1 to 4 minutes on a pan.
3. Fold the tortilla and slice into wedges.

Jicama Salad

Ingredients:

- Place the following in a mixing bowl: 1/2 pound sliced jicama

- sliced fennel bulb and 1/2 sliced small red onion.

Directions:

1. Squeeze a small seedless tangerine over the jicama, fennel and onion mixture.
2. Season with salt and black pepper.

Salmon With Ginger And Sesame

Ingredients:

- Marinate salmon fillet for 15 minutes in the following mixture:

- 2 tablespoons balsamic vinegar

- 2 teaspoon sesame oil

- 1/2 cup soy sauce

- Peeled ginger

Directions:

1. Remove salmon from the marinade and sauté on a hot skillet for about 1 minute on each side.

2. Sprinkle the salmon on sesame seeds.

Pumpkin Soup

Ingredients:

- 1 teaspoon cinnamon powder
- 1/2 teaspoon nutmeg, ground
- 1 cup fat-free milk
- A pinch of black pepper
- 1 green onion, chopped
- 1 yellow onion, chopped
- 1 cup water
- 15 ounces pumpkin puree
- 2 cups low-sodium veggie stock

Directions:

1. Put the water in a pot, bring to a simmer over medium heat, add onion, stock and pumpkin puree and stir.

2. Add cinnamon, nutmeg, milk and black pepper, stir, cook for 10 minutes, ladle into bowls, sprinkle green onion on top and serve.

3. Enjoy!

Spicy Black Bean Soup

Ingredients:

- 2 jalapenos, chopped

- 1 teaspoon oregano, dried

- 1 teaspoon cumin, ground

- 1 teaspoon ginger, grated

- 2 bay leaves

- 1 tablespoon chili powder

- 3 tablespoons balsamic vinegar

- 3 Black pepper to the taste

- 1cup scallions, chopped

- 1 pound black beans, soaked overnight and drained

- 2 yellow onions, chopped

- quarts low-sodium veggie stock

- 2 tablespoons olive oil

- 6 garlic cloves, minced

- 2 tomatoes, chopped

Directions:

1. Put the stock in a pot, bring to a simmer over medium heat, add beans, cover and cook for 45 minutes.

2. Meanwhile, heat up a pan with the oil over medium-high heat, add ginger, garlic and onion, stir and cook for 5 minutes.

3. Add tomatoes, cumin, jalapeno, oregano and chili powder, stir, cook for 3 minutes more and transfer to the pot with the beans.

4. Add bay leaves, cover the pot and cook the soup for 40 minutes more.

5. Add vinegar, stir, cook the soup for 15 minutes more, discard bay leaves, blend the soup using an immersion blender, ladle into bowls and serve with scallions on top.

6. Enjoy!

Shrimp Soup

Ingredients:

- 8 ounces shrimp, peeled and deveined

- 1 stalk lemongrass, crushed

- small ginger pieces, grated

- 6 cup low-sodium chicken stock

- 2 jalapenos, chopped

- lime leaves

- 1 to 4 cups pineapple, chopped

- 1 cup shiitake mushroom caps, chopped

- 1 tomato, chopped

- 1 bell pepper, cubed

- 1 teaspoon stevia

- 1/2 cup lime juice

- 1 cup cilantro, chopped

- 2 scallions, sliced

Directions:

1. In a pot, mix ginger with lemongrass, stock, jalapenos and lime leaves, stir, bring to a boil over medium heat, cover, cook for 15 minutes, strain liquid in a bowl and discard solids.

2. Return soup to the pot again, add pineapple, tomato, mushrooms, bell pepper, sugar and fish sauce, stir, bring to a boil over medium heat, cook for 5 minutes, add shrimp and cook for 3 more minutes.

3. Add lime juice, cilantro and scallions, stir, ladle into soup bowls and serve.

4. Enjoy!

Seafood Stew

Ingredients:

- 1/2 cup shallot, chopped

- 1 cup low sodium veggie stock

- 2 dozen clams, scrubbed

- 1 pound mussels, scrubbed

- 1 Black pepper to the taste

- 1 tomato, chopped

- 8 scallops, halved horizontally

- 2 cups water

- 12 jumbo shrimp, peeled (shells reserved) and deveined

- 4 parsley springs

- 1/2 cup parsley, chopped

- 1 garlic clove, minced

- 1 tablespoon garlic, minced

- 1 tablespoon extra virgin olive oil

Directions:

1. Heat up a pan over high heat, add shrimp shells and 1 garlic clove, stir and cook for 2 minutes.
2. Add parsley springs and water, stir, bring to a boil, cook for 3 minutes, strain into a bowl and leave aside for now.
3. Meanwhile, heat up another pan with the olive oil over medium-high heat, add 1 tablespoon garlic and shallots, stir and cook for 1 minute.
4. Add veggie and shrimp stock, clams and mussels, bring to a simmer and cook for 4 minutes.
5. Divide clams and mussels into bowls, sprinkle chopped parsley and leave aside.
6. Season broth with black pepper, add scallops, shrimp and tomato, cover and cook for 2 more minutes over medium heat.

7. Add this mix to the bowls, sprinkle chopped parsley and serve.Enjoy!

Tuna Kabobs

Ingredients:

- Black pepper to the taste
- 1 tablespoon sesame seeds
- 2 tablespoons canola oil
- 16 pieces pickled ginger
- 1/2 cup low-sodium soy sauce
- 1 pound tuna steaks, cubed in 16 pieces
- 2 tablespoons rice vinegar

Directions:

1. In a bowl, mix soy sauce with vinegar and tuna, toss to coat, cover bowl and keep in the fridge for 35 minutes.
2. Discard marinade, pat dry tuna and sprinkle with black pepper and sesame seeds.

3. Heat up a pan with the oil over medium heat, add tuna pieces, cook them until they are pink in the center and brown on the outside, take off heat and transfer them to a plate.
4. Thread ginger and tuna cubes on the skewers, arrange the kabobs on a platter and serve them with a side salad. Enjoy!

Balsamic Salmon

Ingredients:

- A pinch of black pepper

- 1 tablespoon mint, chopped

- Cooking spray

- 2 pounds salmon fillets, b2 less and skin on

- 1 garlic clove, minced

- 1/2 cup real maple syrup

- 1/2 cup balsamic vinegar

Directions:

1. Heat up a pan over medium-low heat, add maple syrup, vinegar and garlic, whisk, heat up for 1 minutes, transfer this to a bowl and leave aside to cool down.

2. Spray a baking sheet with cooking spray, add salmon fillets, season them with black pepper and brush with 1 of the maple glaze.

3. Introduce in the oven at 450 degrees F, bake for 10 minutes, brush salmon with the rest of the glaze and bake for 20 minutes more.
4. Divide between plates, sprinkle mint on top and serve.
5. Enjoy!

French Style Onion Dip

Ingredients:

- 1 tbsp Worcestershire Sauce

- Black Pepper(ground)

- Olive Oil

- clove Garlic

- 1 cup of low-fat Greek-style Yogurt

- 3 tsp. Kosher Salt

- chopped White Onion

- 2 cup low-fat Sour Cream

Directions:

1. Heat oil in the slow cooker. Sauté the garlic and onion.

2. Add the rest of the elements.

3. Heat on low temp for 30 mins.

4. Garnish with chives (minced). Serve with vegetables.

Turkey, Potatoes & Green Beans

Ingredients:

- 4 Potatoes
- 1 pkg, Smoked Turkey Sausage
- Green Beans (large can)

Directions:

1. Place beans in the slow cooker.
2. Slice the sausages and potatoes and add them to the beans.
3. Pour water to cover the ingredients in the cooker.
4. Stir and cook for 4 hrs.

Chicken And Rice

Ingredients:

- 1 tsp. Chicken bouillon

- Water

- 1 cup uncooked Rice

- lb Mushroom

- 1 lb diced Chicken

- 1 tsp. Poultry Seasoning

- 1/2 tsp sea Salt

- 1 cup chopped Onion

Directions

1. Slice the mushrooms.
2. Grease the skillet with the oil.
3. Sauté the chicken, mushrooms and onion for 15 mins.
4. Add the seasoning and sautéed chicken to the slow cooker.

5. Cook the chicken for 4 hrs. on low.

6. When chicken is partially cooked, add the rice.

7. Cook till the rice is d2   .

8. Serve hot.

Turkey In Mushroom Sauce

Ingredients:

- 1 tsp. Salt

- Pepper

- Mushrooms, sliced

- 1 cup Chicken Broth or White Wine

- 2 tbsp. Corn Starch

- 3 lbs. Turkey Breast (halved and b2 less)

- 2 tbsp. melted Butter

- 2 tbsp. Parsley (dried)

- 1 tbsp. Tarragon (dried)

Directions:

1. Place turkey in the slow cooker. Coat the turkey with the butter.

2. Sprinkle the spices on the turkey.

3. Place mushrooms on top of the turkey.

4. Add wine over the turkey.

5. Heat on "low" temp for 7 hrs.

6. Transfer the turkey to a platter.

7. Now, mix cornstarch with 1/2 cup of water.

8. Add the starch mixture to the slow cooker. Stir well.

9. Boil for 2 mins.

10. Serve turkey with the gravy.

Chicken And Lemon-Filled Tacos

Ingredients:

- 12 Tortillas (wheat)

- 1 cup chunky Salsa Sour Cream

- Mexican Cheese

- Shredded Lettuce

- 1 tbsp. Chili Powder

- Jalapeo

- 2 pounds Chicken Breasts (halved and b2 less)

- 3 tbsp. Lime Juice

- Lemon Zest

- Corn (frozen)

Directions:

1. Place chicken in slow cooker
2. Pour lime juice and chili powder on the chicken Cook on "low" for 6 hrs.

81

3. Transfer the chicken to a platter.

4. Now, shred the chicken.

5. Then add in the corn with salsa.

6. Heat for 30 more mins.

7. Fill tortillas with chicken and remaining ingredients.

8. Serve warm.

Chicken And Green Beans

Ingredients:

- Olive Oil

- 1 tsp. Cilantro (dried)

- Pepper

- Onion Powder

- 2 minced cloves Garlic

- 2 lbs. Chicken Breasts

- 1 lbs. trimmed Green Beans

- 2 lbs. diced Potatoes

- 1 tsp. Oregano (dried)

Directions:

1. Place chicken in the slow cooker.

2. Arrange beans along the sides of the chicken.

3. Next, repeat the process with potatoes.

4. In a bowl, mix all other ingredients.

5. Pour the mix over the arranged chicken, beans and potatoes.

6. Cook on "high" for 4 hrs.

7. Serve.

Tasty Red Beans And Rice

Ingredients:

- 3 celery stalks, chopped

- 3 garlic cloves, minced

- A pinch of black pepper

- 1 teaspoon hot sauce

- 1.5 teaspoon thyme, chopped

- 7 cups water

- 2 bay leaves

- 1 pound chicken sausage, sliced

- 1 red bell pepper, chopped

- 10 cups rice

- 1 pound red kidney beans

- 1 yellow onion, chopped

Directions:

1. In your instant pot, mix the bell pepper with the onion, celery, garlic, kidney beans, black pepper, hot sauce, thyme, water and bay leaves, toss, cover and cook on High for 30 minutes.
2. Add sausage, toss, cover and cook on High for 20 minutes more.
3. Divide the rice between plates.
4. Top each with the beans mix and serve.

Easy Ribs

Ingredients:

- 2 teaspoons garlic, minced
- 1 to 5 cups low-sodium chicken stock
- A pinch of black pepper
- 2 baby back ribs, divided into 4 sections, fat removed
- 1 cup tomato sauce, no-salt-added

Directions:

1. In your instant pot, mix the ribs with the stock, garlic, tomato sauce and black pepper, toss, cover and cook on High for 40 minutes.
2. Divide the ribs between plates, spread the sauce from the pot all over and serve.

Easy Beef Soup

Ingredients:

- 10 baby Bella mushrooms, sliced
- 1 cup yellow onion, chopped
- 6 garlic cloves, minced
- 2 bay leaves
- 1 cup water
- teaspoon thyme, dried
- 2 cups pearl barley
- A pinch of black pepper
- 6 cups veggie stock, low-sodium
- 1 potato, shredded
- 1 to 3 pound beef stew meat, fat removed and cubed
- 1 cup celery, chopped
- 2 tablespoons olive oil

Directions:

1. Set your instant pot on sauté mode, add the oil, heat it up, add beef stew meat, stir and brown for 2 to 5 minutes.
2. Add mushrooms, onions, garlic and black pepper, stir and cook for another 2 to 4 minutes.
3. Add stock, celery, bay leaves, water and thyme, stir, cover and cook on High for 15 minutes.
4. Add potato and barley, stir, cover and cook on High for 1 more hour.
5. Ladle the soup into bowls and serve.

White Bean Stew

Ingredients:

- 1 and 4 teaspoon cumin, ground
- 1 and 3 cups great northern beans, soaked for 12 hours and drained
- 2 teaspoons oregano, dried
- A pinch of black pepper
- 1 and 3 cups water
- 2 cups tomatillos, chopped
- 1 cup poblano, chopped
- 1 cup yellow onion, chopped
- jalapeno, chopped

Directions:

1 In your blender, mix the tomatillos with the poblano, onion, jalapeno and cumin and pulse well.

2   Add this mix to your instant pot, also add the
    beans, water and black pepper, toss, cover
    and cook on High for 40 minutes.

3   Divide into bowls and serve.

Cauliflower Cream Soup

Ingredients:

- 1 pound cauliflower florets

- garlic cloves, minced

- 1 teaspoon sweet paprika

- 1 teaspoon red pepper flakes

- 1 teaspoon thyme, dried

- 2 cup coconut milk

- 4 cups veggie stock, low-sodium

- 1 pound butternut squash, peeled and cubed

- 1 yellow onion, chopped

- 3 teaspoons olive oil

Directions:

1 Set your instant pot on sauté mode, add the oil, heat it up, add garlic and onion, stir and cook for 2 to 4 minutes.

2   Add cauliflower, squash, stock, paprika, pepper flakes and thyme, stir, cover and cook on High for 15 minutes.

3   Add the coconut milk, blend the soup using an immersion blender, divide into bowls and serve.

Chicken Bowls

Ingredients:

- 1 tablespoon chipotle paste

- 1 cup corn

- 2 cup quinoa

- 1 cup water

- Juice of 1 lime

- 1 tablespoon olive oil

- 3 tablespoons cilantro, chopped

- Black pepper to the taste

- 1 cup mild salsa, no-salt-added

- 1 cup cherry tomatoes, halved

- 1 small avocado, pitted, peeled and cubed

- 1 pound chicken thighs, skinless and b2   less

- 3 teaspoon cumin, ground

Directions:

1   In your instant pot, mix the salsa with the cumin, black pepper, chipotle paste, chicken thighs and corn, toss, cover and cook on High for 35 minutes.

2   Transfer this mix to a bowl, clean the pot and add quinoa, water, lime juice and the oil.

3   Toss, cover and cook on High for 5 minutes more.

4   Divide chicken and quinoa into bowls, top each bowl with cherry tomatoes, avocado pieces and sprinkle cilantro at the end.

Tomato Cream

Ingredients:

- 2 carrots, chopped

- 1 tablespoon avocado oil

- 1 cup low-sodium veggie stock

- 1 tablespoon tomato paste, no-salt-added

- 1 tablespoon basil, dried

- 1/2 teaspoon oregano, dried

- A pinch of black pepper

- 1 ounces coconut cream

- 15 ounces tomato sauce, no-salt-added

- 15 ounces roasted tomatoes, no-salt-added

- 3 garlic cloves, minced

- 1 yellow onion, chopped

Directions:

1. In your instant pot, mix the garlic with the onion, carrots, tomato sauce, oil, tomatoes, stock, tomato paste, basil, oregano and black pepper, toss, cover and cook on High for 15 minutes.
2. Blend using an immersion blender, add the cream, toss, divide into bowls and serve.

Thyme Cod

Ingredients:

- 1 can tomatoes

- 2 springs thyme

- 2 cod fillets

- 1 tablespoon olive oil

- 1 red onion

Directions:

1   In a frying pan heat olive oil and sauté onion, stir in tomatoes, spring thyme and cook for 5 to 10 minutes

2   Add cod fillets, cover and cook for 5-6 minutes per side

3   When ready remove from heat and serve

Veggie Stir-Fry

Ingredients:

- 1   cup carrots

- 1/2   cup green beans

- 1 tablespoon soy sauce

- 1 cup onion

- 1 tablespoon cornstarch

- 1 garlic clove

- 1/2 cup olive oil

- 1/2 head broccoli

- 1/2 cup show peas

Directions:

1. In a bowl combine garlic, olive oil, cornstarch and mix well

2. Add the rest of the ingredients and toss to coat

3. In a skillet cook vegetables mixture until tender
   1. When ready transfer to a plate garnish with ginger and serve

Yoghurt & Mango Smoothie

Ingredients:

- 1 cup mango juice

- 2 cup ice

- 1 mangoes

- 1 cup Greek yoghurt

Directions:

1. In a blender place all ingredients and blend until smooth

2. Pour smoothie in a glass and serve

Lime Smoothie

Ingredients:

- 1 lb. mango
- 1 tablespoon milk
- 2 oz. sugar
- Juice of 2 limes

Directions:

1. In a blender place all ingredients and blend until smooth
2. Pour smoothie in a glass and serve

Basil Smoothie

Ingredients:

- 1 handful basil leaves

- 1 cup yoghurt

Directions:

1. In a blender place all ingredients and blend until smooth

2. Pour smoothie in a glass and serve

Peanut Butter Smoothie

Ingredients:

- 1 cup ice
- 1 shot Amaretto
- pinch of cinnamon
- 1 cup milk
- 1 banana

Directions:

1. In a blender place all ingredients and blend until smooth
2. Pour smoothie in a glass and serve

Berry Yoghurt Smoothie

Ingredients:

- 1 oz. vanilla yoghurt

- 1 cup milk

- 1 tablespoon h2   y

- 1 oz. berries

- 2 bananas

Directions:

1. In a blender place all ingredients and blend until smooth

2. Pour smoothie in a glass and serve

Coconut Smoothie

Ingredients:

- 1 cup ice
- 1 tablespoon h2   y
- 1 cup Greek Yoghurt
- 1 cup strawberries
- 2 mangoes
- 2 bananas
- 1 cup coconut water

Directions:

1. In a blender place all ingredients and blend until smooth
2. Pour smoothie in a glass and serve

Kefir Blueberry Smoothie

Ingredients:

- 1   banana (cubed)

- 2   tbsp. of almond butter

- 3   tsps. of 4

- 1   cup of kefir

- 2   cup of blueberries (frozen)

Directions:

1. Add blueberries, banana cubes, and kefir in a blender.

2. Blend until smooth.

3. Add 1 and 2 almond butter.

4. Pulse the smoothie for a few times.

5. Serve immediately.

Ginger Fruit Smoothie

Ingredients:

- 1 cup of water

- Three strawberries

- piece of ginger

- 2 tbsp. of agave nectar

- 1-fourth cup of each

- 3 Blueberries (frozen)

- 1 Green grapes (seedless)

- 2 cup of green apple (chopped)

Directions:

1. Add blueberries, grapes, and water in a blender. Blend the ingredients.
2. Add green apple, strawberries, agave nectar, and ginger. Blend for making thick slushy.
3. Serve immediately.

Fruit Batido

Ingredients:

- 1 can of evaporated milk
- 1 cup of papaya (chopped)
- 1-fourth cup of white sugar
- 1 tsp. of vanilla extract
- 1 tsp. of cinnamon (ground)
- 1 tray of ice cubes

Directions:

1. Add papaya, white sugar, cinnamon, and vanilla extract in a food processor. Blend the ingredients until smooth.
2. Add milk and ice cubes. Blend for making slushy.
3. Serve immediately.

Banana Peanut Butter Smoothie

Ingredients:

- 1 cup of peanut butter
- 3 tbsps. of h1 y
- 3 cups of ice cubes
- 3 bananas (cubed)
- 1 cups of milk

Directions:

1. Add banana cubes and peanut butter in a blender. Blend for making a smooth paste.
2. Serve with banana chunks from the top.

Berry Banana Smoothie

Ingredients:

- 1 banana (cubed)

- 3 cups of vanilla ice cream

- 3 cup of ice cubes

- 3 -third cup of milk

- 1 cup of each

- Strawberries

- Peaches (cubed)

- Apples (cubed)

Directions:

1 Place strawberries, peaches, banana, and apples in a blender. Pulse the ingredients.

2 Add milk, ice cream, and ice cubes. Blend the smoothie until frothy and smooth.

3 Serve with a scoop of ice cream from the top.

Berry Surprise

Ingredients:

- 1 third cup of raspberries

- 3 tbsps. of limeade concentrate

- 1 cup of strawberries

- 1 cup of pineapple cubes

Directions:

1   Combine pineapple cubes, strawberries, and raspberries in a food processor.

2   Blend the ingredients until smooth.

3   Add the frozen limeade and blend again.

4   Divide the smoothie in glasses and serve immediately.

Bruschetta

Ingredients:

- 1/2 whole-grain bread (cut into six 1 " thick diagonal pieces)
- 1 tsp olive oil
- 1 tsp black pepper
- 1 tbsp chopped parsley
- Parmesan Cheese (low fat)
- 2 tomatoes (diced)
- 2 tsp balsamic vinegar
- 2 tbsp basil (chopped)
- 2 cloves garlic (minced)

Directions:

1. Toast flatbread slices until finely browned in an oven at 400 ºF.
2. Mix it with all of the rest of the ingredients.

3. Blend the spoon equally over the toasted
    bread.
4. Topping with a little Parmesan egg.
5. Serve it while it is warm.

Baked Herb-Crusted Cod

Ingredients:

- Cod fillets 4

- 2 tablespoons

- Herb-flavored stuffing 1 cup

Directions:

1. Start by preheating the oven by setting the temperature to 375 degrees Fahrenheit.

2. Take a baking dish and coat it gently with cooking spray.

3. Take a zip-lock bag and add in the stuffing. Seal the bag and crush the stuffing until it is crumbly.

4. Add 1   fillet to the zip-lock bag and coat it evenly with crumbly filling. Keep on a plate. Repeat the process with the remaining fillets.

5. Place the fillets into the prepared baking dish and place the dish into the preheated oven. Bake for 10 minutes.

6. Serve!

Roast Balsamic Chicken

Ingredients:

- Black pepper (freshly ground) ⅛ teaspoon

- Fresh rosemary 8 sprigs

- Balsamic vinegar 1   cup

- Brown sugar 1 teaspoon

- Whole chicken (skinned) 1 (4 pounds)

- Fresh rosemary (minced) 1 tablespoon

- Garlic (minced) 1 clove

- Olive oil 1 tablespoon

Directions:

1. Begin by preheating the oven by setting the temperature to 350 degrees Fahrenheit.

2. Take a small bowl and add in the minced garlic and minced rosemary. Mix well.

3. Place the chicken onto a plate and rub it with the oil and garlic mixture. Nicely sprinkle with freshly ground black pepper.

4. Take 3 sprigs of rosemary and put them into the chicken's cavity. Use butcher's twine to nicely truss the chicken.

5. Take a roasting pan and place the chicken into the same. Place the roasting pan into the preheated oven and roast for around 1 hour and 20 minutes. Baste the chicken after every 15-20 minutes to enhance the flavors.

6. Once the chicken has browned and the juices run clear, take the chicken out of the oven.

7. Transfer the chicken onto a serving platter and set aside.

8. Take a small nonstick saucepan and place it on a low flame. Add in the brown sugar along with the balsamic vinegar and let it heat until the sugar dissolves completely.

9. Carve the chicken and get rid of the skin. Pour the sugar and vinegar mixture over the chicken.

10. Finish by garnishing the chicken with rosemary and serve!

Garlic And Broccoli Rigatoni

Ingredients:

- Olive oil 2 teaspoons

- Garlic (minced) 2 teaspoons

- Black pepper (freshly ground) –as per taste

- Rigatoni (whole-wheat) 1 pound

- Broccoli florets 2 cups

- Parmesan cheese 2 tablespoons

Directions:

1. Take a large pot and place it over a high flame. Fill it more than 1 way and let it come to a boil.

2. Toss the pasta into the boiling water and cook it on high for around 12 minutes or as per package instructions.

3. While the pasta cooks, take a steamer and add the broccoli to the steamer basket. Fill the steamer pot with 2 cups of water. Cover

the steamer basket with a lid and steam for around 10 minutes.

4. Once the pasta is cooked, drain it in a colander and set aside.

5. Take a large glass mixing bowl and add in the steamed broccoli and cooked pasta.

6. Also, add in the parmesan cheese, garlic, and olive oil. Generously season with freshly ground black pepper. Toss well until all ingredients are well combined.

7. Serve right away!

White Broiled Sea Bass

Ingredients:

- Garlic (minced) 1 teaspoon

- Herb seasoning blend (salt-free) 1/2 teaspoon

- Black pepper (freshly ground) as per taste

- White sea bass 2 fillets

- Lemon juice 1 tablespoon

Directions:

1. Begin by heating the broiler and placing the rack at least 4 inches away from the heat.

2. Take a baking sheet and grease it generously with nonstick cooking spray.

3. Place the sea bass fillets onto the baking sheet and season them with lemon juice, herbed seasoning, pepper, and garlic.

4. Place the baking sheet into the oven and broil for around 10 minutes.

5. Serve right away!

Easy Beef Stroganoff

Ingredients:

- Water 1 cup

- All-purpose flour 1 tablespoon

- Paprika 1   teaspoon

- Sour cream (fat-free) 1 cup

- Onion (chopped) 1 cup

- Beef round steak (b1 less) 1 pound

- Yolkless egg noodles (uncooked) 4 cups

- Cream of mushroom soup (fat-free and undiluted) 1 can

Directions:

1. Begin by cutting the beef round steak into slices measuring about 1-inch each. Make sure that you remove all the fat.

2. Take a large cast-iron pan and place it on a medium flame.

3. Add in the onions and sauté until they become translucent. This will take about 5 minutes.

4. Add in the beef and cook for 5 more minutes.

5. Make sure the edges are browned and tender to touch. Drain any excess fat and set aside.

6. Take a large pot and fill it more than 1 way. Place the pot on a high flame and let the water come to a boil.

7. Add noodles to the boiling water and cook for around 12 minutes or as per package instructions.

8. Take a nonstick saucepan and place it on a medium flame.

9. Add in the cream of mushroom soup, flour, and water; stir well and cook for around 5 minutes or until the sauce thickens.

10. Transfer the soup mixture to the beef and mixture; cook on a medium flame until the mixture is heated through.

11. Add in the paprika and stir well. Remove from the flame.

12. Now add in the sour cream and stir to combine well.

13. To serve, place noodles on the plate and top with the soup and beef mixture.

14. Enjoy warm!

Baffle Waffles

Ingredients::

- Sugar 2 tablespoons

- Eggs 2

- Milk (warm) 4 cups

- Butter (melted) 1/2 cup

- Vanilla extract 1 teaspoon

- All-purpose flour 2 cups

- Salt 1 teaspoon

- Baking powder 4 teaspoons \

Directions:

1. Start by preheating the waffle iron to your desired set temperature.

2. Now take a fresh large bowl and add 3 cups of all-purpose flour, 1   teaspoon of salt, four teaspoons of baking powder 1 and 3 teaspoons of sugar.

3. Stir all the ingredients: in the mixture together and keep it aside.

4. Now take a third of a cup of butter and melt it.

5. Now in a fresh bowl take 3 eggs and mix with warm milk, melted butter and 1 teaspoon of vanilla extract.

6. Empty the mixture into the flour mixture and whisk it well to create a slurpy batter.

7. Now grease the preheated waffle iron and pour the batter evenly on it.

8. Close the waffle iron and cook until waffles turn crispy golden.

9. Top the waffle with whipped cream, maple syrup or fruit of your choice and serve hot.

Banana Sour Cream Bread

Ingredients:

- Vanilla extract 2 teaspoons

- Cinnamon (ground) 2 teaspoons

- Salt 1/2 teaspoon

- Baking soda 3 teaspoons

- All-purpose flour 5 cups

- Chopped walnuts (optional) 1 cup .

- Sugar 3 cups

- Cinnamon (ground) 1 teaspoon

- Butter 3 cup

- Eggs 3

- Ripe bananas (mashed) 6

- Sour cream 1 container

Directions:

1. Start by preheating the oven to 300 degrees f (150 degrees c).

2. Take 3 large loaf pans and grease evenly

3. Take a small bowl and add 1   cup white sugar, 1 teaspoon ground cinnamon and stir them together.

4. Now take the cinnamon and sugar mixture and dust spray the greased loaf pans.

5. Take a fresh bowl and add ripe bananas to mash well.

6. In a separate bowl take 3/4 cup of butter and three cups of white sugar.

7. Mix them well.

8. Add three eggs to the same bowl, mashed bananas and mix them well.

9. Now add 16 ounces of sour cream, and 3 teaspoons of vanilla extract and 3   teaspoons of ground cinnamon and stir it well.

10. Add 1   teaspoon of salt, three teaspoons baking soda and four cups of all-purpose flour to the bowl. Stir to make a paste.

11. You can also add walnuts to the paste (optional).

12. Mix them well into the batter. Now evenly spread the batter in the greased large loaf pans and bake well for 1 hour.

13. Insert a toothpick in the center of the pans to check if the bread is baked properly.

14. Cut into slices and serve. Put the remaining bread in the refrigerator.

Cinnamon Baked Bread

Ingredients:

- Brown sugar 1 cup

- Chopped walnuts (optional) 1/2 cup

- Raisins 1/2 cup

- Refrigerated biscuit dough 3 packages

- Sugar 1 cup

- Cinnamon (ground) 2 teaspoons

- Margarine 1/2 cup

Directions:

1. Start by preheating the oven to 350 degrees f (175 degrees c).

2. Take a hard surface 9-inch bundt pan and grease well with cooking spray.

3. Now take a cup of sugar and 3 teaspoons of ground cinnamon in a resealable plastic bag. Mix them well together.

4. Take three packets of refrigerated biscuits dough and cut each dough piece into small quarters.
5. Add at least 8 chopped biscuit dough pieces in the sugar-cinnamon mixture.
6. Seal the plastic bag and shake well until the dough pieces get evenly coated in sugar-cinnamon mixture.
7. Put a layer of sugar-cinnamon coated pieces in the bottom of the greased bundt pan.
8. You can also add chopped walnuts and raisins over the layer to get the crunchy flavor. This step is totally optional.
9. Continue with a layer of sugar-cinnamon dough in the bundt pan.
10. Take a frying pan pour 1 cup of margarine and a cup of brown sugar.
11. Cook the mixture until margarine is completely melted and mixed well with sugar

to form a smooth thick paste. Let the mixture boil for 3   minutes.

12. Now evenly pour the mixture over the biscuit dough placed inside bundt pan.

13. Bake the bread in the preheated oven (350 degrees f) for 35 minutes until it turns puffy and golden brown.

14. Remove the pan and let the bread cool in bundt pan for at least 10 minutes.

15. Once cooled, flip the bundt pan and remove the bread onto a plate.

Buttermilk Pancake

Ingredients:

- Salt 1 teaspoon

- Buttermilk 3 cups

- Milk 1/2 cup

- Eggs 3

- Butter (melted) 1 cup

- All-purpose flour 3 cups

- White sugar 3 tablespoons

- Baking powder 3 teaspoons

- Baking soda 2 teaspoons

Directions:

1. Begin with preheating the to 200 degrees f.

2. In a fresh bowl take three cups of all-purpose, three tablespoons of sugar, three teaspoons of baking powder, 1/2 teaspoons of baking soda, and 2 teaspoon salt and stir it well.

3. Take a fresh bowl, add three large eggs, three cups of buttermilk, 1/2 cup of milk, and 1 cup of butter, and stir them well together.

4. Now empty the mixture in the flour mixture and mix well until the batter turns slightly lumpy. Avoid making it too thin or too thick.

5. Take a large frying pan and heat it on medium flame.

6. Brush the pan with the butter using a scapula.

7. Use 1 cup batter and pour over the hot pan. Turn the batter upside down with a spatula once each side is evenly golden brown in color.

8. Remove the cakes on a plate and transfer them in the preheated oven to stay warm.

9. Use the remaining batter to make cakes.

10. Once cooked, serve hit with maple syrup or spread of your choice.

French Toast With Blueberries

Ingredients:

- Vanilla extract 1 teaspoon

- Maple syrup 1 cup

- White sugar 1 cup

- Cornstarch 2 tablespoons

- Water 1 cup

- Blueberries 1 cup

- Butter 1 tablespoon

- Day-old bread 12 slices

- Cream cheese 2 packages

- Fresh blueberries 1 cup

- Eggs 12

- Milk 2 cups

Directions:

1. Take a 9x13 inch baking dish and evenly grease it with cooking spray.

2. Now cut 12 slices of day-old small bread into 1 -inch cube each.

3. Take 1 of the sliced bread cubes in the baking dish

4. Now cut 3 eight once of packages of creamed cheese into 1-inch cubes and put those nicely over the layer of arranged bread cubes in the baking dish.

5. Take 1 cup of fresh blueberries and sprinkle them over bread cubes on cream cheese.

6. Top the blueberries with remaining pieces of bread cubes. Now take a fresh large bowl, break 12 eggs into it, and beat nicely. Add 3 cups of milk, 1 teaspoon of vanilla extract and 1 cup of maple syrup in the bowl with beaten eggs. Now mix all the ingredients: together.

7. Take the mixture and pour evenly over the cubed bread mixture.

8. Ensure that the bread cubes are nicely dipped in the liquid mixture.

9. Now cover the mixture with an aluminum foil and refrigerate the mixture overnight. Remove the bowl from the refrigerator at least 1 an hour before baking the next day. Now preheat the oven to 350 degrees f (175 degrees c).

10. Put the baking dish in the oven and bake for 30 minutes.

11. Now remove the aluminum foil from the baking dish and bake for another 30 minutes. Now take a fresh pan and add a cup of sugar, 3 tablespoons of cornstarch, and 1 cup of water.

12. Mix the solution and boil while continuously stirring the mixture. Cook for at least 3 minutes.

13. Mix a cup of fresh blueberries to the heated syrup and simmer the haet as the blueberries begin to burst and leave color.

14. Add 1   tablespoon of butter in the mixture and pour the blueberries sauce over the baked toast.

15. Cut into pieces and serve with maple syrup or the blueberries sauce.

Plump Pumpkin Bread

Ingredients:

- Baking powder 1/2 teaspoons

- Baking soda 2 teaspoons

- Salt 2 teaspoons

- Cinnamon (ground) 2 teaspoons

- Nutmeg (ground) 2 teaspoons

- Cloves (ground) 2 teaspoons

- Canned pumpkin puree 3 cups

- Vegetable oil 2 cups

- Sugar 4 cups

- Eggs 6

- All-purpose flour 4 cups

Directions:

1. Start by preheating the oven to 350 degrees f (175 degrees c).

2. Now take three 9x5 inch loaf pans and grease them using regular cooking spray.

3. Evenly spray all-purpose flour pan on the greased loaf pans and set them aside.

4. Now take a fresh large bowl and add 6 eggs into it. Beat them gently into a paste.

5. Add three cups of canned pumpkin puree, 1 cups of vegetable oil, and four cups of sugar in the bowl with beaten eggs and mix well to form a thick paste.

6. Now take a big bowl and add 4 cups of all-purpose flour, 1teaspoon of baking powder, 1 teaspoon of baking soda, and 1 teaspoon of salt, 1 teaspoon of ground cinnamon, 1 teaspoon of nutmeg, and 1 teaspoon of ground cloves.

7. Whisk all the ingredients: together and add to the pumpkin paste. Stir the mixture until it is evenly blended.

8. Now place the batter evenly in the greased loaf pans.

9. Once 1 , put the greased loaf pans in the preheated oven and bake for at least 50 minutes.

10. Use a toothpick inserted in the center of the dish to check if it is properly baked or not.

11. Remove the loaf pans from the oven and let it cool for 15-20 minutes.

12. Cut into slices and serve with creamed cheese or nuts of your liking.

Vintage Pancakes

Ingredients:

- Salt 1 teaspoon - sugar 1 tablespoon
- Milk 2 cups - egg 1
- Butter (melted) 3 tablespoons
- all-purpose flour 1   cups
- Baking powder 1   teaspoons

Directions:

1. begin by taking 1 cups of all-purpose flour in a big fresh bowl.
2. Add 3 teaspoons of baking powder, 1 teaspoon of salt, and 1 teaspoon of sugar into the flour bowl.
3. Now create space in the center of the flour mixture and pour 2 cups of milk, 1   egg, and three tablespoons of melted butter.
4. Mix all the ingredients: together until you get a smooth batter.

5. Now take a medium frying pan and heat it spraying a little oil over it.

6. Take a quarter cup full f batter and spread over the medium heated frying pan.

7. Spread the batter evenly without leaving any lumps.

8. Heat the cake until the sides start turning golden brown.

9. Flip the pancake using a spatula once you see little bubbles on the surface of the cake.

10. Serve the pancakes hot with a topping of your choice or maple syrup.

Baked Chicken Breasts

Ingredients:

- 2 cups chicken stock

- 2 teaspoon tarragon, chopped

- 1 cup white rice

- 1 to 3 cups white wine

- 2 cup wild rice

- 1 to 3 cups celery, chopped

- 1 pound chicken breast halves, skinless, b1 less and cut into medium pieces

- 1 to 3 cups pearl onions

Directions:

1. Put 1 of the stock in a pot, add chicken, tarragon, onions and celery, stir, bring to a simmer over medium heat, cook for 10 minutes, take off heat and leave aside to cool down.

2. In a baking dish, mix the rest of the stock with white and wild rice, stir and leave aside for 30 minutes.
3. Add chicken and the veggies, cover, introduce in the oven at 300 degrees F and bake for 1 hour.
4. Divide between plates and serve right away.
5. Enjoy!

Roasted Chicken

Ingredients:

- Black pepper to the taste

- 1 cup balsamic vinegar

- 1 teaspoon stevia

- 8 rosemary springs

- 1 whole chicken

- 1 garlic clove, minced

- 1 tablespoon rosemary, chopped

- 1 tablespoon olive oil

Directions:

1. In a bowl, mix garlic with rosemary and stir.
2. Rub chicken with black pepper, the oil and rosemary mix, put it in a roasting pan, introduce in the oven at 350 degrees F and roast for 1 hour and 20 minutes basting with pan juices from time to time.

3. Meanwhile, heat up a pan with the vinegar over medium heat, add stevia, stir and cook until it dissolves.
4. Carve the chicken, divide it between plates and serve with the vinegar mix drizzled all over.
5. Enjoy!

Chicken Salad And Peanut Dressing

Ingredients:

- 1/2 cup low-sodium peanut sauce

- 1 napa cabbage head, shredded

- 2 cup carrot, grated

- 2 scallions, sliced

- Black pepper to the taste

- 1 teaspoons sesame seeds

- 3 cups chicken, cooked, b1 less, skinless and shredded

- 1/2 cup olive oil

- 1 cup rice wine vinegar

- 2 teaspoons sesame oil

Directions:

1. In a bowl, mix olive oil with peanut sauce, vinegar and sesame oil and whisk very well.

2. In a salad bowl, mix chicken with 4 scallions, cabbage and carrot.
3. Add peanut dressing and pepper and toss to coat.
4. Divide between plates, sprinkle sesame seeds and the rest of the scallions on top and serve.
5. Enjoy!

Braised Brisket

Ingredients:

- 1 pound celery, chopped

- A pinch of salt

- Black pepper to the taste

- 1 cups water

- 1 pound sweet onion, chopped

- pounds beef brisket

- 1 pound carrot, chopped

- 8 earl grey tea bags

For The Sauce:

- 1 pound sweet onion, chopped

- 8 earl grey tea bags

- 1 tablespoon stevia

- 1 cup white vinegar

- 16 ounces canned tomatoes, chopped

- 1 pound celery, chopped

- 1 ounce of garlic, minced

- 2 ounces olive oil

Directions:

1. Put the water in a pot, add 1 pound onion, 1 pound carrot, 1 pound celery, salt and pepper, stir and bring to a simmer over medium-high heat.

2. Add beef brisket and 8 tea bags, stir, cover, reduce heat to medium-low and cook for 7 hours.

3. Meanwhile, heat up a pan with the oil over medium-high heat, add 1 pound onion, stir and sauté for 10 minutes.

4. Add garlic, 1 pound celery, tomatoes, stevia, vinegar and 8 tea bags, stir, bring to a simmer, cook until veggies are 1 and discard tea bags at the end.

5. Transfer beef brisket to a cutting board, leave aside to cool down, slice, divide between

plates and serve with the sauce drizzled all over.

6. Enjoy!

Veggie Stir Fry

Ingredients:

- 1 red bell pepper, cut into medium wedges

- 1 yellow bell pepper, cut into medium wedges

- 2 garlic cloves, minced

- 1 zucchinis, cut into medium wedges

- 13 ounces baby corn, halved

- 1 small broccoli head, florets separated

- 2 tablespoons low-sodium veggie stock

- 1 cup low-sodium soy sauce

- 2 tablespoons cornstarch

- 2 tablespoons stevia

- 1 tablespoon ginger, grated

- 1 yellow onion, chopped

- 2 tablespoons olive oil

Directions:

1. In a bowl, mix the stock with the soy sauce, cornstarch, stevia and ginger and whisk well.
2. Heat up a pan with the oil over medium-high heat, add the onion, stir and cook for 1-2 minutes.
3. Add red bell pepper, yellow bell pepper, garlic, zucchini, corn, broccoli and the cornstarch mix, stir, cook for 8 minutes, divide into bowls and serve.
4. Enjoy!

Mexican Quinoa Mix

Ingredients:

- 2 red bell peppers, chopped

- 2 pound chicken meat, ground

- 1 cups low-sodium tomato sauce

- 1 cup canned kidney beans, drained and no-salt-added

- 3 ounces low-fat cheese, grated

- 1 cup quinoa, dry

- 2 cups low-sodium veggie stock

- 1 tablespoon olive oil

- 2 red onions, chopped

- 2 garlic cloves, minced

Directions:

1   Put the stock in a pot, add quinoa, bring to a simmer over medium heat, cook for 20 minutes and take off heat.

2   Heat up a pan with the oil over medium-high heat, add onions and garlic, stir and cook for 1 to 5 minutes.

3   Add bell pepper, chicken and quinoa and toss a bit.

4   Add tomato sauce and kidney beans and toss again.

5   Sprinkle the cheese all over, introduce the pan in the oven and cook at 360 degrees F for 20 minutes.

6   Slice, divide between plates and serve.

7   Enjoy!

Belgian Endive Chicken

Ingredients:

- 3 diced heads Belgian Endive

- 2 minced Bacon Strip

- 2 sliced tart apples

- 1 cup unsweetened Apple Juice

- 1 pounds Chicken Thighs (skinless and b1 less)

- 2 tbsp. Caraway Seeds 1/2 tsp. Kosher Salt

- Ground Black Pepper

Directions:

1   Rinse and pat dry the chicken.

2   Season the chicken with pepper ,caraway seeds and salt.

3   Roll up the thighs.

4   Place them on the bottom of the slow cooker.

5   Now, arrange a layer of endive in the slow
    cooker.

6   Spread the Bacon strip evenly on the endive.

7   Add a layer of Apple slices.

8   Add apple juice to the slow cooker. Cook on
    "low" for 6 hrs.

9   Serve the chicken on heated plates.

Artichoke Chicken

Ingredients:

- 2 minced cloves of Garlic

- Balsamic Vinegar (white

- 2 sliced leeks (green and white)

- 2 ounces Artichoke Hearts

- 2 cup Chicken Broth or White Wine

- 1 tsp. Paprika

- 1 pounds Chicken Pieces (skinless and b1 less)

- Olive Oil

- Cayenne Pepper

Directions:

1. Season the chicken with Cayenne and paprika.

2. Sauté chicken pieces for 2 mins in oil.

3. Transfer the chicken to the cooker.

4. In same pan, cook leeks, vinegar and garlic for 1 min.

5. Add the artichokes along with broth or wine.

6. Transfer them to slow cooker.

7. Heat on "low" temp for 6 hrs.

8. Enjoy!!!

Peppered Cod

Ingredients:

- 1 pounds Cod filets

- Lemon Zest

- 2 tbsp. Balsamic Vinegar

- Olive Oil

- Black Pepper(cracked)

Directions:

1. Divide a foil paper into 1   big portion and 4 small packets.

2. Use pepper, lemon zest and vinegar to coat the fish.

3. Wrap the fish with the foil tightly.

4. Cook on "high" for 2 hrs.

5. Serve hot.

Chicken In Italian Sauce

Ingredients:

- 1 chopped yellow Onion

- 2 tsp. Italian Seasoning

- 1 oz. diced Tomatoes (unsalted)

- 1 cup Red wine

- Black Pepper (. Ground)

- 1 oz. Chicken Breast (skinless and b1 less)

- Olive Oil

- 1/2 tsp. Kosher Salt

- clove Garlic

- 2 green Bell Pepper

Directions:

1. Coat the chicken with pepper and salt.

2. Sauté chicken in oil for 6 mins.

3. Transfer the chicken to a plate. In slow cooker, pour 1 tbsp. olive oil and heat on

"high." Sauté bell pepper, garlic and onion for 5 mins.

4. Add the tomatoes.
5. Cook on "low" for 2 hrs.
6. Cook continuously for next 20 mins but uncovered.
7. Add the chicken.
8. Heat again on "low" temp for 2 hrs.
9. Serve immediately.

Sesame Salmon Fillets

Ingredients:

- 2 skinless Salmon fillets

- Salt

- Black Pepper(ground)

- 1 Sesame Oil

- 2 tbsp. Vinegar

- 1 tsp. Sesame Seeds (black) 1/2 tsp. Ginger (ground)

Directions:

1. Coat the slow cooker with oil. Set the cooker on "high".
2. Place the salmon in the cooker. Drizzle the sesame seeds, pepper, salt and ginger on the salmon.
3. Turn after 3 mins and repeat the procedure.
4. Add vinegar and cook on "high" for 20 mins.
5. Transfer the salmon to a plate. Serve immediately

Rice With Chicken And Veggies

Ingredients:

- 1 cup red bell pepper, chopped

- garlic cloves, minced

- 2 teaspoon ginger, grated

- 2 cup edamame beans

- 2 cup carrots, grated

- 4 cups water

- A pinch of black pepper

- 1 cup white rice

- 4 cup coconut aminos

- 1 chicken breast, skinless, b1 less and cubed

- 1 cup broccoli florets

- 3 cup rice wine vinegar

- 4 teaspoons arrowroot powder

- 2 tablespoons olive oil

Directions:

1. In your instant pot, mix the aminos with the vinegar, arrowroot powder and oil and whisk well.

2. Add chicken, bell pepper, black pepper, cloves, ginger, carrots, rice, water, broccoli and edamame beans, cover and cook on High for 20 minutes.

3. Stir the whole mix once again, divide it into bowls and serve.

Simple Chili

Ingredients:

- 2 tablespoons tomato paste

- 1 teaspoon cocoa powder

- 1 tablespoon avocado oil

- 1 yellow onion, chopped

- 3 garlic cloves, minced

- 1 tablespoon chili powder

- 1 tablespoon cumin, ground

- 1 teaspoon oregano, dried

- A pinch of black pepper

- 1 pound chicken meat, ground

- 1 cup low-sodium chicken stock

- 2 cups corn

- 2 ounces canned kidney beans, no-salt-added, drained and rinsed

- 3 ounces canned tomatoes, no-salt-added

Directions:

1. In your instant pot, mix the stock with tomato paste, cocoa powder, oil, onion, garlic, chicken, chili powder, cumin, oregano, kidney beans, tomatoes, corn and black pepper, toss, cover and cook on High for 15 minutes.

2. Divide the chili into bowls and serve.

Carrot Soup

Ingredients:

- 1 yellow onion, chopped

- 2 tablespoons cilantro, chopped

- 1 to 3 cups veggie stock, low-sodium

- 1 tablespoon red curry paste

- 12 carrots, chopped

- 14 ounces coconut milk

- 2 garlic cloves, minced

Directions:

1. In your instant pot, mix the carrots with the garlic, onion, milk, stock, curry paste and cilantro, toss, cover and cook on High for 15 minutes.

2. Blend using an immersion blender, ladle into bowls and serve.

Lentils Soup

Ingredients:

- 1 celery stalk, chopped
- 3 garlic cloves, minced
- 1 teaspoons cumin, ground
- 1 teaspoon turmeric powder
- 1 teaspoon thyme, dried
- 1 cup brown lentils, rinsed
- 2 ounces baby spinach
- 5 carrots, chopped
- 3 cups veggie stock, low-sodium
- 2 teaspoons olive oil
- 4 yellow onion, chopped

Directions:

1. Set your instant pot on sauté mode, add the oil, heat it up, add onions, celery and carrots, stir and cook for about 5 minutes.

2. Add garlic, cumin, turmeric, thyme, lentils and stock, cover and cook on High for 12 minutes.

3. Add spinach, cover, cook on High for 3 minutes more, ladle the soup into bowls and serve.

Easy Chicken Cacciatore

Ingredients:

- 1 chicken legs

- 16 ounces canned tomatoes, no-salt-added and chopped

- 2 tablespoons avocado oil

- 1 yellow onion, chopped

- 3 carrots, chopped

- 1 cup chicken stock, low-sodium

- 2 red bell pepper, chopped

- 1 pound mushrooms, sliced

- 3 garlic cloves, minced

- 1 teaspoon oregano, dried

- 1/2 teaspoon red pepper flakes

- 1/2 cup balsamic vinegar

- 1 tablespoons basil, chopped

- 2 tablespoons parsley, chopped

- Black pepper to the taste

- 1 teaspoon thyme, chopped

Directions:

1 In your instant pot, mix the chicken with black pepper, oil, onion, carrots, bell pepper, mushrooms, garlic, oregano, pepper flakes, basil, stock, tomatoes, vinegar and thyme, toss, cover and cook on High for 20 minutes.

2 Add parsley, toss, divide between plates and serve.

Sweet Paprika Pork Chops

Ingredients:

- 1 tablespoon olive oil

- A pinch of black pepper

- 1 teaspoon sweet paprika

- 1 cup chicken stock, low-sodium

- 4 pork chops, b1 less

Directions:

1   Set your instant pot on sauté mode, add the
oil, heat it up, add pork chops, brown for a
few minutes on each side, add paprika, black
pepper and stock, cover the pot, cook on High
for 5 minutes, divide between plates and
serve.

Simple Pork Roast

Ingredients:

- 4 pounds pork shoulder

- 1 tablespoon olive oil

- 1 cup beef stock

- 1/2 cup Jamaican spice mix, no-salt-added

Directions:

1   In a bowl, mix pork with oil and spice mix and rub well.

2   Set your instant pot on sauté mode, add pork, brown for a few minutes on each side, add stock, cover the pot and cook pork shoulder on High for 40 minutes.

3   Slice roast and serve

Broccoli Cream

Ingredients:

- 1 cups low-sodium chicken stock

- 1/2 teaspoon garlic powder

- 1 cup carrots, chopped

- 2 tablespoons olive oil

- 1 yellow onion, chopped

- A pinch of black pepper

- 1 broccoli head, florets separated and roughly chopped

- 1 cup coconut cream

- 3 cups fat-free cheddar cheese, shredded

Directions:

1   Set your instant pot on sauté mode, add the oil, heat it up, add onion, stir and cook for 2-3 minutes.

2   Add carrots, broccoli, stock, garlic powder, salt and pepper, stir, cover, cook on High for 5 minutes, add cream, blend using an immersion blender, ladle into bowls, sprinkle cheese on top and serve.

Coconut Chicken Mix

Ingredients:

- 1 cup white onion, chopped

- 1 tablespoon water

- 1 tablespoon ginger, grated

- 2 teaspoons coriander, ground

- 1 tablespoon lime juice

- 1 teaspoon cinnamon, ground

- 1 teaspoon turmeric powder

- 1 teaspoon fennel seeds, ground

- Black pepper to the taste

- 3 tomatoes, chopped

- 14 ounces coconut milk

- 1 pounds chicken thighs, skinless, b1 less and cubed

- 1 red chilies, chopped

- 2 tablespoons olive oil

- 1 cup low sodium chicken stock

- 2 garlic cloves, minced

Directions:

1 In your food processor, mix white onion with garlic, chilies, water, ginger, coriander, cinnamon, turmeric, fennel and black pepper and blend until you obtain a paste.

2 Set your instant pot on sauté mode, add the oil, heat it up, add the paste you made, stir and cook for 30 seconds.

3   Add chicken, tomatoes and stock, stir, cover the pot and cook on High for 15 minutes.

4 Add coconut milk, stir, cover the pot again and cook on High for 7 minutes more.

5   Add lime juice, stir, divide into bowls and serve.

Coconut Matcha Smoothie

Ingredients:

- Three tbsps. of white beans (drained)
- 1 tbsps. of shredded coconut (unsweetened)
- 1 tsp. of matcha green tea (powder)
- 2 cup of water
- 3 large banana
- 1 cup of frozen mango cubes
- 1 leaves of kale (torn)

Directions:

1. Add cubes of mango, banana, white beans, and kale in a blender.
2. Blend all the ingredients until frothy and smooth.
3. Add shredded coconut, white beans, water, and green tea powder.
4. Blend for thirty seconds.

5. Serve with shredded coconut from the top.

Cantaloupe Frenzy

Ingredients:

- Three tbsps. of white sugar

- 3 cups of ice cubes

- 1 cantaloupe (seeded, chopped)

Directions:

1. Place the chopped cantaloupe along with white sugar in a blender. Puree the mixture.
2. Add cubes of ice and blend again.
3. Pour the smoothie in serving glasses. Serve immediately.

Berry Lemon Smoothie

Ingredients:

- 1 cup of blueberries

- 1 third cup of strawberries

- 1 tsp. of lemonade mix

- Eight ounces of blueberry yogurt

- 1 to 3 cup of milk (skim)

- 1 cup of ice cubes

Directions:

1 Add blueberry yogurt, skim milk, blueberries, and strawberries in a food processor. Blend the ingredients until smooth.

2 Add lemonade mix and ice cubes. Pulse the mixture for making a creamy and smooth smoothie.

3 Divide the smoothie in glasses and serve.

Orange Glorious

Ingredients:

- 1 cup Milk

- 1 cup of white sugar

- Twelve ice cubes

- 2 tsp. of vanilla extract

- Six ounces of orange juice concentrate (frozen)

- 1 cup of each

- 2 cup Water

Directions:

1. Combine orange juice concentrate, white sugar, milk, and water in a blender.

2. Add vanilla extract and ice cubes. Blend the mixture until smooth.

3. Pour the smoothie in glasses and enjoy!

CPSIA information can be obtained
at www.ICGtesting.com
Printed in the USA
BVHW050844020622
638737BV00014B/292